I0407028

I AM...
Bigger Than Your
Work Injury

Tanya Nelson

Book Illustration by Jourdyn Montgomery

ISBN: 1540481859
ISBN-13: 978-1540481856

DEDICATION

This book is dedicated to all the injured workers. As I have spoken with others in their struggles during their work injury, each one is different. One has contemplated suicide, one has struggled emotionally, mentally, psychologically, and physically, others have given up because of the long battle. I say, "Thank You" for standing even when the war against you seems like you are outnumbered. Thank you for not giving up as you push forward and rebuild on broken pieces of life.

You can do it!! Live and share your story.

CONTENTS

Acknowledgments

Introduction 5

1 My Story Begins 7

2 Physical Therapy 9

3 The Tug of War 12

4 Injection Day 15

5 Lawyer on My Side 17

6 Company Doctors and Therapy 18

7 The Fight to Keep Me at The First Clinic 22

8 The Gates of Hell Will Not Prevail 27

9 A New Road Ahead? 34

10 The Lies Begin 38

11 The Letter That Changed Everything 44

12 Closing the Middle 53

About the Author

Acknowledgements

I acknowledge Yahweh, Yeshua, and the Holy Spirit. I have heard Him speak to me more since the work injury than any other time in my life. I would not be who I AM and where I Am if it was not for the Yahweh. I love You All.

Thank you to my kingdom fiancé, Andrew Samuel for believing in me. You came into my life at a time when Abba knew my walk with Him was first. We have prayed, cried, laughed, studied, and completed each other. I love you Honeybunny! ☺

Thanks to my family who has been there for me through love, growth, inspiration, perseverance, longsuffering, my times of complaining, times of couch surfing, and times of transitioning. I love you and thank you each for pouring into my life.

I would like to acknowledge my friends. Yahweh brought you all in at different times, but the time was relevant. Some of you were with me during my time in Egypt, others were with me crossing the Red Sea, some made it to the mountain, and others crossed over with me where I am now. There are many to name so, I must say, Thank You to each one of you for your heart, your ear, your faith when I was in doubt, your trust when I didn't know who to trust, and your time that is valuable. I love you all and together we can change Wrongs to Rights.

Thank you, Regina Baker for believing in this book, for encouraging me to believe in myself and to walk in the purpose Yahweh created in me. I look forward to the release of the next 2 books with you, Ms. Baker, as I know you will push me beyond my reach. I love you Sister and thanks a million.

INTRODUCTION

Remembrance

As I sat in the clinic today (November 2, 2015), I remembered at the end of my conversation with the neurosurgeon that it has been one year today since I injured my back at work. Sitting, waiting on the doctor, the Holy Spirit, the third person of the Godhead, began to encourage me by reminding me of Yahweh's most powerful, all-inclusive name revealed to us in Genesis 15:1, which is "I AM". I AM .... your source, I AM .... your healer, because of My (Yahshua) stripes you were healed. Isaiah 53:5

I AM that I AM .... who sees every secret meeting held and every idle word spoken against you and I AM that I AM .... who wants you to forgive those who wronged you, so you can be forgiven and set free."

I AM... BIGGER Than Your Work Injury

Yahweh really is bigger than anything that is before you. Yahweh wants to expose the enemy behind the curtain of the Worker Injury system that keeps honest people from getting the help they deserve.

The Holy Spirit asked me to write a book on my experience with Workers Injury, so what follows is a result of my obedience. I will start from the beginning.

1-MY STORY BEGINS

On November 2, 2014, I went to empty the trash gondola, which could weigh up to 40-175 lbs. with cardboard. The freezer gondola could weigh up to 300lbs once it is full.

There are two cardboard compactor doors and inclines on both sides. You must push the trash gondola up one incline, get a running start to push it down and up the other incline, and angle it towards the compactor door. I knelt, grabbed the grab bar, pulled up on it, and felt a sharp pain in my lower back that radiated to the front of my lower stomach. I could not rise due to the shaking/spasm that I was experiencing. When I finally rose up, I tried to shake off the pain, and tell myself that I would be alright. I knew I had to report it to my supervisor immediately and I did. I tried to work through my shift, but the pain became unbearable. I spoke with my supervisor about leaving and letting me rest my back through the night.

On my drive home, I thought about water as hot as I could stand it to relieve the pain. I tried the hot water, but it did not help, so I went to bed. The next day my supervisor called to check on me, and I dropped the cell phone on the floor. I was screaming to my supervisor, "I dropped the phone, give me a minute to pick it up, please! My supervisor was concerned about me and had spoken to the night Senior Manager about what happened. My supervisor (Allison) said, "We spoke to HR, and it might be something far more serious. Please come in and fill out the paperwork so you can have your back checked out. I went up later that night and completed all the necessary paper work about the accident.

Allison said there was a Baylor Hospital up the street, and I could go there. They would have to drug test me also based on company policy. I went to Baylor and spoke with the night ER guy about my back and he said they could X-Ray it, but he was not able to drug test me. I told him my supervisor said I must be drug tested. I called Allison while leaving and she said just go to Contra Clinic in the morning.

I went to Labcorp to do my drug test, so it would be completed in the allotted timeframe. I left from Labcorp and drove to Contra Clinic for my X-rays. Contra Clinic looked at my paperwork and said you must go to Ova Medical. I drove to Ova Medical where they checked me in and did an X-Ray. The X-Ray revealed that I had a bilateral sprain to my lumbar and abdominal spasm to my lower stomach. I told Dr. Stan that my pain was a 7 which was high to me.

He placed me on pain and inflammation medicine, set me up with physical therapy, and gave me restriction paperwork returning to work the next day. I have listed some solutions that would help you out from the beginning of an injury.

Solutions of Help

A. If you don't say your pain is a 10 in the beginning they will only do an X-Ray instead of a MRI. If you think something is seriously wrong, specify a 10.

B. Watch the wording on your paperwork concerning your injury. It can be confusing and misleading.

C. If you can take someone with you, do so.

D. You can pick a doctor to treat you and not your company's Doctor.

E. Make sure you are not driving under the influence of medication even if they say it's alright to do so.

F. If they schedule your physical therapy or doctor's appointment during your work hours, there is a form the doctor must complete so you can be reimbursed for those hours.

G. Stick with the same Doctor. They will try to switch up on you.

H. Whenever you are given Work Restriction Paperwork, always have them to explain everything to you. If they specify hours on your paperwork for that body mechanic, ask questions. For example: Does this mean light lifting for one hour in eight hours worked or one hour and a break?

I. Always remember that it is your body part that is injured.

J. If they are sending you back to work and you know something is wrong, ask them to take you off work. If the doctor says, they cannot take you off work, file a complaint with the Worker's Injury System, the insurance company website, Better Business Bureau, YELP, etc. This informs other injured workers about your previous experience with this clinic or the doctors.

2 – PHYSICAL THERAPY

I went across the hallway to their physical therapy area. I spoke to the physical therapist and she did a physical check of my back after completing the questionnaire. I left from Ova and took the paperwork to Allison (my supervisor). She told me not to come in until next week because I was still barely moving. I asked her to use my vacation time, so my check wouldn't be so short. I received a call from the insurance company to check on me and to send me paperwork to fill out about the injury.

I was released to do light therapy that same week to help my back. My first day to therapy was rough. The therapist had me to do light body mechanics to stretch my back muscles. It was very painful.   I did as much as my back would allow.

I went back to the doctor for a follow up the next week, and he released me to do light duty work and three days of physical therapy. I took my restriction paperwork in and gave it to my supervisor. A copy of my work restrictions, along with the rest of the paperwork, and other doctor visits will be on my Facebook page for Targeted Individuals for you to review. The light duty work consisted of: quality assurance of customer orders, checking locations for expired medication, stocking the A-frame locations for production, and counting inventory.

After a couple of weeks of therapy, my physical therapist had me to do a box weight that I was hesitant to do in the first place.   We had worked up to me lifting 25lbs., but we did not do it consistently.   The box weight is a wood box that is designed to hold weights.   I told her, "No." She said you did 25lbs. the other day so let's increase. I said yes hesitantly. It was 40lbs with 1 repetition of 5. I completed all my therapy for the day and left to run an errand for my grandmother. The pain was worse and now with a burning sensation in my lower back. I let them know the next day at therapy about my symptoms. They did electro therapy and ice to see if it would help. It did not help me at all.   I overheard the head therapist say she needs to stay for at least 1 1/2 hours. I called off to work that day.

 I had an appointment with Dr. Stan (company's doctor) the next day and he made notes into the computer system about what happened during therapy. I told him my back was burning now, but he didn't do much except document. I went back in to work after being off a day and could not get through 4 hours before the pain and burning intensified.

I left from work and went to the hospital because the burning was scaring me. The ER didn't do much after I told them it was a work injury. She pressed my back and I screamed, but, I wanted to knock fire from her. She apologized and said, "I'm so sorry I didn't mean to push so hard." She told me to continue to follow my treatment with the Workers Injury doctor and if it gets worse to come back to the ER. You are treated differently when it is a work injury.

I continued to complain about the pain and the burning as I went into therapy and work. This went on for three weeks before the approval of a MRI. I finally got a MRI in December 2014 at an imaging clinic across from the doctor's office. They did a MRI on my lower back and said it would be ready in 24-48 hours. Each day I went to therapy I would ask about my MRI and they would tell me it's not in yet. I called the imaging place and she said I faxed it over last week. I knew something was not right. I asked for the lady to fax it again, and I would let the clinic know. It took one and half week before the MRI was read to me. I came in for therapy and asked again about my MRI reading and my therapist said, "Yes it's in and it shows that you have disc herniation L4-5, S-1. I told my therapist, "You all thought I was not being truthful about my back, but I know something was wrong." She said, " I never doubted what you were saying."

 I noticed, while on vacation, that if I stayed settled and on the heating pad, my pain would decrease some. I went back for a follow up with (New Company Doctor) Dr. Britain and asked him if he could take me off work. He said, "Worker's Injury doesn't like for us to take people off work." I begin to question him about the work restriction paperwork and the body mechanics I was performing. I was lifting, twisting, bending, stooping, and standing longer than what was on the restriction paperwork.

I said, " When I come in here and tell you I did twisting, turning, and bending all night what did everyone think?" I told Dr. Britain they need to explain this to people because I shouldn't have been working, and my supervisor wouldn't have accommodated the restrictions. Dr. Britain said, "Yes we have to do a better job of explaining the restrictions to everyone." I asked Dr. Britain to explain what my MRI meant, and he said, "The insurance is going to see if they can fix it by giving you injections first and then possible surgery." I said, what is the injection for?" He said, "This is to help with inflammation and pain. Dr. Britain processed my request for a consultation with a Neurosurgeon. One of my neighbors had some work done on her leg and referred me to this clinic in Arlington, Texas. I turned that information in to the front desk as a referral, and they believed the insurance would allow me to use that clinic.

FOOD FOR THOUGHT ON THERAPY!

A). Physical therapy is there to rehabilitate you back to health, but often they are pushing to get you released back to work too soon.

B). Some of the therapist pretend to be concerned about you, but others genuinely care.

C). I would hear the therapists gossiping about patients after they had left physical therapy for the day.

D). When you complain about something you are closely monitored.

E). Be persistent and honest about your treatments.

3 – THE TUG-OF-WAR

I went visit with the Neurosurgeon, Dr. Wake in January 2015. He looked at my MRI and said, you would never need surgery, but I think an injection should fix your back issue." He did a referral for me to see Dr. Kai. I went to the Orthopedic doctor for a consultation, and he spoke to me about getting an injection in my lower back. Dr. Kai said the insurance is only going to approve one injection and it is like an act of congress to get a second one. I agreed to the injection and asked Dr. Kai if he could release me from work until after the injection. Dr. Kai said, He could not release me from work because he was not my administering doctor. My job could not accommodate my restrictions, but they did not want this to hit their safety number. I was only making my back worse by trying to do the work, and now I was put in a tug-of-war. It was the company's safety number, the insurance, and my bills.

CHAIN OF EVENTS

1.   I was asked to come in and do filing with a lower back injury on Jan. 6, 2015 after my manager said he had nothing in his department.

2.   On Jan 9, 2015 Orthopedic doctor put me down for No kneeling, bending, squatting, and stooping. Another department supervisor still had me to come in and do a sit-down job where I would access the construction guys into the cage area.

3.   I was told on Jan. 14, 2015 that I couldn't keep leaving early and needed to go back to my doctor. I told Amy that I was under the influence of Tramadol on this day.

4.   After being given the run around about releasing me from work on Jan. 14, 2015. Dr. Britain modified my restrictions because of my pain. He said the specialist would have to release me. Dr. Britain informed me that WC doesn't like for them to take people off from work.

5.   On Jan. 15, 2015 I asked Dr. Kai after the consultation to release me and he said, "Your administering doctor (Dr. Britain) will have to release you." He was the doctor who was prescribing my medication.

6.   The therapist noticed how inflamed my back was on the 15th of January and did some lower back massages and shock therapy.

7.   On Jan. 16, 2015 I received $56.59 for the 2 weeks runaround! I still had not received anything from WC. I spoke with Risk Management about what was going on with my back, still going in to work, and my pay. I was stressed out now, but trying to hold it together.

8.   On Jan. 16, 2015 I spoke with Amy and told her what the new restrictions read, and she said her offer still stood with the 2 hours of sitting. I explained to her my pain issue and how would I drive if the doctor said No standing and No walking? Amy replied, "How do you go to the rest room? I told her I would go and then get back in the bed on my heating pad.

9.   On Jan. 19, 2015 I saw Dr. Britain when I was leaving therapy and he thought they had released me from work based off the new restrictions. I am still thinking; these people have my best interest at heart. His concern, was all an illusion.

10.   On Jan. 21, 2015 I was told the first group of construction guys would be finished and there would be no more work until Jan 27, 2015. Amy said to come in, and she would find something for me to do.

11.   On Jan. 21, 2015 Dr. Wake released me from work until my injection approval through W/C was approved. I called his nurse crying about my back, and she said he would take me off until then.

NOTE: Whenever they take you off work it speeds up the approval process through the insurance company. I made it to the clinic and she forgot that she had spoken to me the day before about releasing me. I faxed a copy over to the claim adjuster and took a copy to Tom (Night Senior) on Jan. 21 of my updated paperwork stating that Dr. Wake had taken me off work.

- Whenever you are taken off work for 7 consecutive days, they must pay you through W/C. When this happens, it means you move up the progressive ladder with the insurance company.

- They really want you to get frustrated and give up.

- Whenever the claims representative calls you for your statement and they tell you it is being recorded, please write all the questions down you want answered in advance. Always answer truthfully. If you got questions regarding treatment, doctors, or pay ask during these recordings. They will try to use it against you later during a hearing.

- Print out all email correspondence between the claims representative and yourself.

- If your claims representative is denying doctor's request or not responding to calls or email, file a complaint against them to the (Your State) Department of Insurance.

4 – INJECTION DAY

Dr. Kai scheduled the injection for February 9, 2015. I received all the paperwork from the insurance quickly about what had been approved. I checked into the Spine Hospital and I was called back shortly where Dr. Kai and his team had me to lie on my stomach while he administered the injection. I felt a sharp stick in my spine and then pressure. The nurse asked how I was feeling. She told me to take it easy.

When I got in the car, I thought what did I allow to just happen?

Below is what I experienced after the steroid injection.

Symptoms/Experiences After Injection

1). Feb. 9, 2015 - Blood pressure 177/107- after the procedure I felt bad. I got into the car, and I could barely keep my seat belt buckled because of the pain.

I took 5 tramadol that day. I itched throughout the night, and I had pressure on the right side under my belly button. I went to the restroom in the middle of the night.

2). Feb. 10, 2015 - I am still in pain, still sitting more on the left side, not able to bend backwards or raise arms overhead, and I had to get up to go to the restroom in the middle of the night.

3). Feb. 11, 2015 - I am still in pain, walked to mailbox and pain in the same spot, still using restroom in the middle of the night.

4). Feb. 12, 2015 - I still have pain in my lower back, still not able to bend backwards, raising arms overhead hurts. Later, that morning I went to Sam's warehouse with a friend and I noticed my pain had never left and sharp pains were also on the left side. I had to hold onto a couple of the poles to get through that experience. They called from the Ortho office to set up the next back injection consultation for Feb. 19 at 11 am and physical therapy at 4:30 pm. When I made it to the 2:30 appointment with Dr. Britain, my blood pressure was 171/101. He said to make an appointment with my primary doctor about my blood pressure. Later, that night my head was hurting me so bad that it felt like it was about to burst.

The same day after my visit with Dr. Britain, I made an appointment with my primary doctor regarding my blood pressure being elevated. He wrote me a prescription for my blood pressure. I was taking medicine for my back and blood pressure now.

5). I went to a follow up with Dr. Wake on Feb. 13, 2015 where he released me to return to work with restrictions.

6). On Feb. 15, 2015 - I went to church for 1 1/2 hours and my pain is at a 6 and my head is hurting.

7). On Feb. 16, 2015 - I went back to work overseeing the construction site again and it was a struggle. My claim's adjuster sent me an email to see if I was back at work or not? I sent her a reply letting her know that I was there and not lifting anything.

8). On Feb. 17, 2015 - I was reevaluated at physical therapy. They changed my appointment from the 18th to the 17th. My blood pressure was high. The therapist had to take it three times. When this happens, the therapist must get the approval of Dr. Britain for me to do therapy. She took out some rehab equipment, but let me leave the weights on to do hamstring curls, knee high lifts, and a sobriety walk. She stayed with me the whole time. She asked me questions about the injection, what did my primary care say, and had my pain increased?

9). On Feb. 19, 2015 - Follow up with Dr. Kai
I refilled out all documents pain lower back...most 6, lowest 4, average 5, it was a 5. Pain was both sides, he said the injection probably hadn't taken effect yet, and he gave me Lyrica 75mg. I told him about sweating at night, pressure on bottom right stomach, and headaches. Dr. Kai said it was from the side effects.

10). The month of Feb. 2015, 2016, and 2017 has come and gone, and still no menstrual cycle. Did the injection sterilize me or was the back injury such trauma on my back that it completely stopped my menstrual cycle?

5 – LAWYER ON MY SIDE

1). A lawyer is only paid a percentage of your work injury benefits. For example, your total benefit payout is $573 a week. The lawyer is paid $125 and the $448 is owe to you.
2). They will see what you don't see.
3). They take a lot of the stress of the insurance off you.
4). They will check to see if you are compensated correctly.
5). They will question if the insurance denies something.
6). They keep you informed of the next step to take.
7). They will go to hearings with you also.

Later, that night while everyone was sleeping I pondered over my previous conversation with my aunt and what she said about how I had been treated throughout this entire process. I did some research and came up with a law firm out of Houston. You will read a little bit about them in a letter I mailed out to several organizations concerning the Worker's Injury system, but they too have a process to follow. I later apologized to them regarding what I had written about them in my letter, which I will share later.
I filled out the information on line and received a call from one of the lawyers the next day. William explained to me some of the processes about Worker's Injury and how they will be compensated. I was excited to know I had help on my side. A young lady was sent to my house later that day with paperwork for me to sign. I spoke with my lawyer about changing doctors, my current treatment, all my questions, and about my pay checks that had been shortened since my injury. They walked me through the process of changing doctors. They questioned anything that was denied, recovered $4500 that had been shortened from my paychecks, and explained to me the designated doctors' visits, etc.

I can say from experience that if you fight it alone it will become stressful and overwhelming.

6 – COMPANY DOCTORS AND THERAPY

During my visit at Ova Medical, they would on occasion, move people away from because they would share with me the things that they had been going through since coming to the clinic. I know they lost this lady's paperwork and had her transferred to several clinics. She had herniated disc to her L1-L5 lumbar, and S-1 damage. She could not feel her toes and had to be driven by her daughter and work light duty. Between lost paperwork for MRI and the transfer to multiple clinics, it hindered her progress. Our appointment days were changed, and I no longer saw her anymore. One lady had been at therapy for over one year and needed surgery for carpal tunnel. Before I transferred to the new clinic she was still there doing physical therapy. Typically, people don't want to get involve with WC because it is robbing the patients out of proper treatment, but lining the pockets of the insurance companies, doctors, therapists, and pharmaceutical companies.

On Feb. 20, 2015 while at therapy I did what my back would tolerate during therapy.

I went to therapy today and had some indirect statements made that only pertained to me. Dr. Nicki asked me how I was doing, and I said, "fine in a low voice." She said you just said, "You are here?" I later told her that was not what I said, I told her I replied, "I am doing fine just my back." The head therapist was in also.

Dr. Nicki came and asked me if I was wearing the weights today on my ankle. I told her, after I left on Tuesday my lower back was bothering me. That is when Dr. Krush said to the head therapist (Daniel), "How is it you can do something one day, but you can't do it again when you return the next time? I don't understand people. I wish I could sit on them (the head doctor said, or be mean like her.)

I was lying on the table and couldn't see who she was referring to. Later, when I went to do rows against the wall, all three of them were close by and the Head therapist said smile. Dr. Krush stood close by as she pretended to take a picture. I don't mind them watching me as I improve my back to recovery, but there is zero tolerance for that type of professionalism.

19

I really felt they were on my side, but I started seeing early signs that they were trying to get my pain down and keep me at work. The focus now is the pain. They began moving people that would share their stories away from me. I would be the last person on schedule for therapy.

I sent my lawyer an email about what I had encounter at the therapy clinic today.

On Feb. 24, 2015, Vanessa (AOA W/C personnel) called me today and left a message concerning my physical therapy. I returned her call and left her a message because she didn't answer. She is over the worker's injury department for Arlington Orthopedics Associates. She called me back and made small talk about the weather and staying warm. She then asked what was going on with physical therapy. I said, "I am still going to therapy." I explained to her I had told the physical therapists that I couldn't do the stuff that had 00 restrictions on it. I told Dr. Britain and he said to let them know in physical therapy and they would make the necessary adjustment.

She said, "Are you still at Ova Medical?" I replied, Yes! She said she would let the claim representative know because they had not turned anything in.

She also said Dr. Kai told her he wasn't requesting another injection, and did he explain to me why? I let her know he needed my pain level down to a three before he could do another injection. I told her he started me on Lyrica. Since, I had her on the phone I asked her about the EMG concerning the nerve damage that Dr. Wake had requested, and Britain was following up on. I told her my claim representative sent me a sheet for what I was approved for and that was it. She said she would follow up on that.

I sent my lawyer an email letting her know that I had spoken with Vanessa and should I discontinue communicating with her. My lawyer (Monifa) said to not speak with her and to let them know I had legal representation and they could speak with her (Monifa).

On Feb. 25, 2015 I made it to therapy and could feel all eyes were on me. This type of bullying is on another scale. It's different from work place bullying. It's done very low-key and under handed by professionals.

David (the therapist assistant) asked what my pain level was, and I smiled and told him a 4. I remembered what Dr. Krush had said about me last

Friday. I asked her if she would check my blood pressure and she did. She squeezed the gauge several times. I felt my pulse beating fast. She told me my blood pressure was 170/93. I began to pray when she instructed me to go to the table and rest for 10 minutes to get it down.

I went to the table and laid down, but I really wanted to speak to her. She took it a second time and it was still high. She asked for me to lie on the table again and to think happy thoughts. I finally stopped her and said, "Dr. Krush you are a physical therapist whose responsibility is to rehab people during their recovery period." I told her that she said some horrible things about me on Friday that was not appropriate, and I must forgive her for that. She said, "What did I say so I can correct it?" I said, "Don't worry about it, I forgive you."

I went back to the table to lay down, but could still feel the tension in the room. The head therapist (Daniel) was there, Dr. Nicki, Dr. Krush, David, and the new guy. I went to the treadmill and then headed back to the table to do my stomach exercises.

I could feel their eyes on me as David told me what to do. Dr. Nicki told me she would have to do my observation. I said cool. I got through all my exercises, and I began to do the rows and my back was hurting. Dr. Nicki said, "Tanya are you doing ok." I said, "No Doc, my back is hurting. "She said, what made it hurt?" I said it is hurting. She said, "Was it the marching?" I said, " No, I think it was the weights."

Dr. Nicki did my observation which included: range of motion, going forward and backwards was still not good, side-to-side was 50/50. I asked her about twisting and why did it hurt? She said, "When you are crossing over to get stuff, it is causing movement with those discs which can cause you to be more inflamed." She said, "You don't want to twist on those discs. "She iced my back down with shock. I told her I wanted to speak with her when I finished. She sat on the bed next to me, but I told her not now wait until the end of therapy.

She took all my stuff off, and I asked her to go to the desk where everyone was. I told them on Saturday, I did my Sabbath and that there was a spirit of deceit, control, and gossiping here. I asked them to forgive me if I said or made them feel any type of way. I also apologize about slamming their door on last Friday. I spoke and said we will have to give account to Yahshua for every thought and word spoken one day. I gave them a recap of all I had gone through since being injured. I have been injured since Nov. 2, 2014, I didn't get an MRI until December 2014, and I got an injection in February 2015 based on results of MRI from December 2014. I have worked since then and did therapy. I told Dr. Nicki since she is the only one that helps, I needed another MRI. I know yawl get people playing games, but I am injured. Dr. Daniel said, "No, we give people the benefit of the doubt." I told them all, I am serious about my back. I am trying to do therapy, but my back is bothering me. I am tired of being in pain and I want it fixed. I don't want to go into the summer with my back like this. I felt like that was weight off my shoulders because I said what was on my heart.

7 – THE FIGHT FOR ME TO STAY

On March 4, 2015 I thought I had good news, but later found out that Vanessa got me into this clinic. They focus on your pain only. There are thirteen procedures (experimental treatments) that they do before they even consider surgery. I wrote this to my lawyer:

Good Evening, I just wanted to say, "Thank You." I am confident that my back will receive proper treatment now. I went to Wolmint today and met with Dr. Stephens. He has scheduled me for a full evaluation on March 11, 2015 at 9:30 am. I was scheduled to see Dr. Britain on yesterday, but had to reschedule it for March 9, 2015 due to inclement weather in Texas. Is there anything that can be done to prevent a gap in my time?

I was now going to two clinics at the same time. Jay told me as she checked the system that the insurance had paid their invoice and they were also paying Ova Medical for seeing me. I wanted out of Ova Medical. They did not do right medically towards my back, and was not persistent for my treatment during this injury.

On March 13, 2015, I called Ova for them to release all my medical information to Wolmint Clinic, so I can begin physical therapy. They said they had not received anything for medical release. I called Jay at Wolmint and she said she sent all my forms on March 6, 2015 and everything takes five business days to be approved. They are trying to see if the insurance would approve more therapy. Jay said, "Your lawyer might have the paperwork and he can fax it to us, so we can start your therapy." The form is a DW53. I let Jay know that I have a follow up with Dr. Wake on the March 20th and Dr. Kay on March 24th. I have an EMG scheduled with Wolmint on April 1, 2015(Which was cancelled by the insurance company).

Later, that day, I checked the mailbox and received a denial letter regarding my request to change treating doctors. The reason for denial is stated as is:

The information provided did not show sufficient justification to support approval. A subsequent request may be made by submitting a new DWC FORM-053, Employee's Request to Change Treating Doctor-Non-
Network, with additional supporting documentation, to the TDI-DWC for consideration.

Other: Box 21, Please provide supporting documentation or release letter from current treating doctor. Also, Box 2, SSN information on form 53 does not match information in DWC records.

I also received a REQUEST FOR DESIGNATED DOCTOR EXAMINATION

TO DETERMINE MMI, IR, DISABILITY, AND RTW.

I didn't understand any of this and sent an email to my lawyer to ask the following questions and if they were still my representatives? How did my SSN get entered into the system incorrectly?

Do I go back to Ova Medical on Monday to see Dr. Britain and Physical therapy?

Your lawyers are still your legal representation and will walk you through the stress of both letters. What I learned from both situations: Do not stop treatment with the other clinic until you have received an approval letter for change of treating doctor. You never want gaps to be showing in your treatment. Make sure they have entered all your information in the W/C system correctly. Follow up, follow through, and follow up again.

A). Don't leave or cancel any appointments until all your request to change doctors has been approved.

B). The state will send you a letter letting you know if you were approved or denied.

C). Pick a doctor of your choice after you have done proper research.

D). They will send you back to the doctor you are trying to leave if the request has not been approved.

On March 20, 2015 I checked to see if my lawyer received my fax on yesterday.

What do I do with that paperwork? Do I need to have anyone to sign it and send it back to Austin? I had the front clerk from Ova Medical letting me know that I could not keep changing my treating doctor. They had not received anything to release me to Wolmint, so I was still on stand-by. I let my lawyer know I was having sharp pains periodically go down the crack of my butt and up my back, pressure on my lower back, with my pain at a 4, my menstrual cycle has been off since this whole ordeal and completely stopped, sweating every night, constipation, and frequently urinating. I began to drag my right foot to decrease some of the pain off my back. I asked my lawyer to expedite my concerns.

We went back and forth for four days trying to get me back into the clinic, so I could see a doctor and get medication. The clinic said the insurance hadn't sent anything and the other clinic was still pending.

On March 21, 2015, my aunt was visiting from Austin on spring break and I asked her to go with me to my appointment. She is on my list for emergency contact. I was first checked in by a nurse who thought I was new to their office. She wrote everything down on this sheet that I told her regarding my pain, medication I am currently taking, side effects I am experiencing, and what had been done so far. The Physician Assistant to Dr. Wake came in next to see what was going on and talked about a diabetes test for my blood, and if I was pregnant since weird things were happening with my cycle. I told her No I wasn't pregnant because I was abstinent from sex. I also told her my primary doctor had already done blood work and nothing came back about diabetes.

I asked if I could have another MRI and she said due to the cost, insurance companies won't pay for another one unless it's been a year since the other one. Dr. Wake came in next and said, "Your pain has improved some, but still some pain. He said, "Your pain is a 4/10." I told him my pain was 4/6 which was my highest pain level since coming there. He then said what a 4 is to you might be a 10 or a 1 to someone else.

My aunt and I could tell he was not happy with me. He said, "I don't think you need surgery, but it's up to you when you see Dr. Kai on whether or not to get the second injection, I am leaving that up to you. He started filling out and changing things on my Worker's Injury sheet that was already filled out. He said I am going to leave you lifting 25lbs, but still 0 bending, kneeling, or squatting. He said, "Are you still on light duty?" I said yes, "I am not lifting anything I am watching the construction guys." I also told him about my experience with my Granny while grocery shopping this past month and the pain I was in. He said, "I will change it to 20lbs and I believe in 4 weeks you can return to work full duty." I told him I couldn't lift that. He said, "There is no reason for me to see you back in my office, I am finished with you and you ladies can leave my office and have a good day."

The lady asked me and my aunt to go around to the other window to be checked out. My aunt was talking to me about the rudeness of the staff and how he basically brought me in today to dismiss me. My aunt said yes the doctor could lift 25lbs because he is 6'5 and about 230lbs. The clerk looked over my paperwork and asked for me to sign off on my worker's injury paperwork. I told her I could not lift that. She said, you must sign because he has already filled it out. I did as she told me to and left.

I sent my lawyer an email that same day to let her know what happened at the clinic today, check on the status of me going to Wolmint, and to get approval for my EMG.

I did a follow up with Dr. Kai about my injection on Tuesday, March 24, 2015. I told him I had pressure on my lower back, frequent urination, constipation, and had missed menstrual cycle for the month. He said the Lyrica was probably causing the issues with my bowel and urine. He said the disc could be pressing against something causing other issues. Dr. Kai said, make an appt with your primary doctor as soon as possible. He set me up for a follow up in 6 weeks, stopped the Lyrica, and put me on Gabapentin. I called my primary doctor's office on March 25, 2015 to explain to them the issues I was having. The nurse said the earliest they could get me in was in May. I still had an appointment for my annual on the 14th of April. Teisha (My primary physician's assistant) said for me to go to the ER and have them to fax everything over or bring it on the 14th when I come in.

A friend of mine drove me to the ER in Arlington. I was going to the restroom ever 15-30 minutes on the hour. They did an X-ray on my bladder. Due to my blood pressure being up they did an X-ray on my chest too. The doctor said I was having bladder spasm and he didn't know what was causing them. They gave me a prescription for tramadol and phenazopyridine.

While at the ER my friend witnessed them putting me in a room and forgetting about me for hours. Someone had erased my name off the board as if, I had been discharged. The ER doctor that saw me went home at 10 pm and another doctor came in unaware of what was going on. The ER doctor said he was called in from North Richland Hills hospital to work the ER in Arlington. My friend said, If I wasn't here tonight I wouldn't believe this myself. It was weird because I had never experience that before at the hospital. It's like something strange happens when you tell them it is a work injury. I sent my paperwork into my lawyer, so they could send it to the claim adjuster for payment.

Things to Remember:

A). Read your discharge paperwork before signing it.
B). Make sure the diagnosis for what you describe is correct.
C). Always forward it to the insurance or lawyer for payment.

8 – THE GATES OF HELL WILL NOT PREVAIL

On April 3, 2015, I went to my appointment for a Functional Capacity Evaluation(FCE) in Dallas, which was ordered by the state.

When I received the paperwork, it scared me in the beginning. It said if you were not being truthful you could be fined or imprison. I knew my back was still messed up and there was no way I could go back to my manual job right now. I begin to fill out the paperwork as the Holy Spirit spoke and said fill out everything that pertains to you. Don't be intimidated because you are being truthful. If your pain ranges from one number to another, explain that in detail on the paperwork. I filled out everything that applied to the injury. I made mention of how I felt while trying to do light duty and while doing normal task away from work.

I went to the clinic, signed in, and sat until they called me back. When the doctor came in my heart begin to beat fast because I instantly thought about my last experience with my aunt and I at the Arlington Clinic. I went into prayer and I felt one million warrior angels with me during that prayer.

I got a peace that I never experienced, and I knew it was the presence of Yahweh's peace. The doctor did an examination on my body mechanics, and asked if I had any questions that hadn't been answered. This was my opportunity to be heard because he was documenting everything.

A). Write down any questions you need answered

B). Share your treatments from other doctors since he is documenting what you are saying.

C). Relax, meditate, and eat before the appointment.

D). This is done for the insurance.

E). Pray

F). Second part to the FCE is your Physical ability is tested next.

G). You might call in to work after the testing. I missed 3 1/2 days due to pain and burning.

The first part of the FCE test take approximately 45 minutes to one hour. The FCE doctor will answer any questions that have gone unanswered during your treatment. He or She will also document your concerns about the treatment you have received prior to visiting the FCE doctor. This doctor will also make final determinations about your impairment rating. You will see this individual 2-4 times over a two-year period. The FCE doctor appeared to be the most honest during my interaction with doctors in the W/C system.

Below are emails corresponding between my lawyer and I during April - May 2, 2015. Maybe some of the answers to questions that have been pressing you are in the emails below.

On April 10, 2015, I still did not have a treating doctor and was out of medication. I was back on my regular shift at work and they placed me on the over-flow line. Dr. Wake had released me to do 20lbs. I was standing outside an assembly line that housed totes that were overflowing with orders. Once these totes come in to me, I was responsible for straightening the product inside the tote and then push it on the flow through line. While working this line some of the totes were heavier than 20lbs. If I did not have any totes on the line, I had to check the product on the shelves for expired dates. All of this was bothering my back. Since I don't have a treating doctor right now, what do I do about medications?

My lawyer response:

Dr. Britain is still allowed to treat you, so you can go back to him. I'm going to follow up on this switch and push it through. I will let you know when it gets approved.

Myself:

I called Ova Medical Clinic and they still have not heard anything. What is the hold up with Wolmint Clinic? Can I go to them? I am in a lot of pain and they have me lifting totes and pushing them off on the over-flow line. I need help, please.

My lawyer response:

What is Ova waiting on? They are treating doctors they don't have to wait for anything, they can just see you. Wolmint switch is pending.

Myself:

I am at Wolmint today seeing Dr. Stephens. He gave me medications the last time I saw him. I called Ova again on yesterday to make an appointment and they scheduled me for tomorrow at 11:15 am. Jay said they are paying for my visits to Wolmint. Do I still go to Ova on tomorrow or should I cancel it? I need an updated WC restriction paperwork for the job by tomorrow. I will ask Dr. Stephens for one today and if he can't give me one due to the holdup of the state DW-53 form, I will have to see Dr. Britain correct? Let me know, please. I had my annual yesterday with my primary Doctor and, he said the issues with my cycle and bowels need to be filed with WC. He gave me a list of testing that need to be done before they do a MRI on the front area of my lower stomach. An Estrogen test for progesterone, estrogen, FSH, testosterone, and LVH. I will let Dr. Stephens know today.

My lawyer response:

The switch has not been approved, I have requested a release from care from Dr. Britain but have not received it. You can reschedule tomorrow's appointment so that we can get more time to get this switch approved. We don't want you to cancel simply because it may send the wrong message (you don't wish to treat) which is not the case you just don't want to treat with them.

Myself:

Ok, no problem. I will be there at 11:15 am.

On April 16, 2015, I went to Ova today and mentioned the following issues to Dr. Britain's nurse. Sharp pain and burning in my lower back and pain that radiates from my lower back to the front on my upper right thigh. I tried telling her about the Estrogen test and she said to let Dr. Britain know.

My blood pressure was 152/98, and she asked if I had coffee or an energy drink. I told her my blood pressure was up due to my pain. I asked her to keep typing and she said to tell Dr. Britain the rest when he comes in. Dr. Britain spoke briefly with the nurse outside and then went into the office and made a call.

When he came in, he asked How I was doing? I told him not good. He said, "What's wrong?" I said she put it in the system. He said, "Let me look and see." He looked over everything that the assistant placed in the system. I told him about my Estrogen Test that needed to be done because my primary said it was due to my injury. He said WC is not going to cover it because they are going to say it could be due to your stress level. I said I haven't had this issue in the past and I have seen my doctor since I was 18. He said, "Your doctor should have seen you for that." I said, "No, it was due to my injury. My blood pressure is up, and I guess that's not due to my pain." He said, "Yes that could be due to your pain." I asked about my

EMG and he said, "They still have not done that?" I said, "No, I am constipated, and I want a MRI for my stomach and hip area." He said they would have seen those issues with your stomach during the MRI. I told him, no because they were focusing on my back. My hip area had been bothering me since the injection. Dr. Britain said to speak with my claims representative. I said, "She won't speak to me because I have a lawyer." He said, "What is your lawyer working on for you?" I replied, to change my treating doctor because I need someone to be aggressive about getting my back to where it was. He shifted the conversation to my claim representative. " He said, "Oh, if your claim representative is denying all your stuff you might need to do like one of my other patients did and speak to her supervisor and change claim representative." He told me I needed the EMG done and if approved for the Estrogen Test, they would locate someone in the network. He said the FCE just updated my information but need me to complete the rest of the test (which is tomorrow). He asked about the Ortho doctor and why Dr. Wake released me last month. I gave him a copy of those restrictions. Dr. Britain said, no follow up with Wake. I said, "No, because he was not happy about me bringing someone else into the office during my last visit." It was my Aunt who is my emergency point of contact. I believe he thought she was someone else." He was very unprofessional. He asked when was I going back to see Dr. Kai and I told him on the 5th of April. He took me off Tramadol due to my bowel issue and kept me on Flexural, Motrin, and something for constipation. I was scheduled for 6 rounds of therapy starting Monday and a follow up with him in 3 weeks. He had me to do the flex bending for movement. It hurt bending over, backwards, and even twisting. I told Dr. Britain, I am not a patch job and I need my back fixed. I got a lawyer because I have no voice.

Dr. Britain asked me if Dr. Wake put 20 lbs. on my restriction paperwork? I responded, " Yes, and he shook his head.

I emailed my lawyer after speaking to Dr. Britain about removing Tam Johnson (claim representative) off my case so I can get my EMG, MRI, and Estrogen Test approved and done. Let me know your thoughts?

My lawyer response

On April 17, 2015, Dr. Britain gave you wrong information, you cannot switch claim representative. A claim representative switch is done is when the claim representative leaves for some reason or another (promotion, fired, dept. change, etc.). He needs to sign the release from care, so we can get you over to Wolmint. I have sent him the request we are pending his response.

During the week of April 20-22, 2015, I sent several emails in the same day to my lawyer regarding my treatment, changing doctors, and the denial letters from the state. If you do not hear from your lawyer, keep communicating with he or she as things change.

Myself:

I was waiting on the pending response to change from Ova to Wolmint. I went to the second part of Exam Works with the FCE. I am in a lot of pain. It was a 5 when I left but it is very well a 7-8 without meds. She said she would send her part out to the insurance and employer, along with my copy. Will they send you a copy or not?

My lawyer's response:

Sometimes but not always. I ask for an update file copy from your insurance carrier every 2 months.

Myself:

I can send it to you when they send it to me. They sent me another denial letter on my DW-53 form again on yesterday.

My email to my lawyer regarding Dr. Britain

I go to the clinic (April 20-22) this week for therapy. Would you like for me to have a conversation with him regarding my DW-53 form? This form allows you to change treating doctors. He has lied several times about things.

He is covering up me lifting the 40lbs box weight, I had no burning, and no sharp pain until the box weight happened. Why would they let me lift that much weight with herniated disc? They claim they did not have my MRI reading for 1 1/2 week. Now he was holding on to my paperwork for me to change treating doctor.

Let me know what to do or should I just keep quiet?

Myself:

On April 20, 2015, they reevaluated me at therapy today. I asked Dr. Britain to tell me what he placed in my file after my last visit with him. He just requested paperwork from Dr. Wake and Kai. Dr. Britain never asked for another MRI, an EMG, or an Estrogen Test. I will print the doctor release from treatment form and have Dr. Britain to sign it tomorrow.

My lawyer's response on April 20, 2015

Yes, tell him you want to see another doctor and need the release from care signed, I have attached a copy to this email.

Myself:

Are you able to correct the information on it? I could not edit the other client's information because it was a protected document. I got my copy from the lawyer printed out and took it to Dr. Britain to sign.

I asked Dr. Britain to sign my release paperwork for me to see another doctor. He said no problem. When I finished up with him and made it to the front desk, the administrative lady was trying to schedule my next appointment and therapy. I told her I was released as of today. She gave me my Restriction paperwork, prescriptions, and told me good luck.

I felt a lot of pressure was off my shoulders now and could move forward with good treatment. In route home the front desk admin called and said, "Dr. Britain would like to set you up with an FCE appointment. I told her I did one of those during the beginning of April and was awaiting the documents from it. Why would they offer this to me now? I had been at their clinic since the injury. I will put a copy on the Targeted Individual Facebook page.

My lawyer response:

I already sent the release from care, so it takes 7 days to get it approved. Call Dr. Wake and confirm they've resubmitted the DW- 53, I will do the same.

Myself:

On April 30, 2015, I did my MMI on April 3, 2015 in Dallas. Dr. Lamb (State Doctor FCE) is supposed to report his findings in 7 business days after the examination. Has he sent anything to you because I haven't received anything. I did the second part of the FCE in Bedford on April 17, 2015 and have not heard anything from them. Who fills out the DWC Form-069? I am asking because it is listed on the back of my old appointment sheet with Dr. Lamb.

My lawyer response:

Because of the FCE they get an extension on the 7 days rule. Your report is not due until May 15, 2015. It will be sent out to you, me, the Division, the insurance, and your treating doctor, who is Dr. Britain at this point.

Myself:

I receive a letter today!

My lawyer response:

What letter?

Myself:

From the Disability Determination Office. I also got a call from someone at Broadspire today. I did not answer it. I will fax over a copy to you tomorrow. I believe he is advising them to remove the disc. Should I return the call to Broadspine or wait until after you review everything, and you can speak with them. I am at work now and must clock in.

On May 1, 2015, an individual with Broadspine name Betty Knows call and left me a voice message. She said she was a claim manager calling to check on the status of my medical condition and that she would be in the office until 4:30 pm today. She said Tam Johnson is no longer on the case.

I sent my lawyer an email letting her know what my response was to the voicemail message from Betty Knows. I would like the surgery to fix the entire issue. I also want an Estrogen Test done for my Cycle, EMG done for my nerve damage, and a MRI done on the front lower right side of my stomach/hip area where the pain radiates from my back. She asked how I was doing. In pain (elevates from a 4 to a 6 while working) back burning (lifting, pushing, or reaching over in the totes to do date checks), sharp pain (While standing and pushing off totes from the overflow line), and lifting more than the 10lbs Dr. Lamb (State Doctor FCE) put on the W/C sheet. I will fax everything over to you. Can you speak to Betty on my behalf after you review the fax?

My lawyer response:

Did you let her know you were represented? There should be no reason anyone from the insurance contacts you directly. For future situations let them know you have an attorney, have a great day.

Myself: I did not speak to her, she left a message. The insurance company already know I have legal representation.

9 – A NEW ROAD AHEAD?

On May 5, 2015, I went to my final visit with Dr. Kai today in Arlington. I know my lawyer told me not to cancel any appointments. AOA did not email me or leave a message concerning the appointment like they did in the past. Did they want me to miss this last follow up?

When I made it to the window to check in the young lady said, she showed up.

One of the women went and spoke with Dr. Kai and he went to the back of the building. I checked in with Dr. Kai's nurse about the pain in my lower back and radiating on the right-side hip. I also mentioned my menstrual cycle again. I told her my pain is a 4 on meds. She said he will be in.
Dr. Kai came in and said, "I see you are still having problems with your cycle." I said, "Yes." He said, "Did you get with your OBGYN?" I said, "Yes." He (My primary) said he is not getting involved because it is WC and that once I start paying, they will charge me for everything. He said that's not true. He needed to check to make sure everything else was alright.

You're not pregnant, are you? I said, "No he did a pregnancy test for my annual. I am not having sex." He said, "Did it stop after the injection? I said, "Yes it completely stopped after the injection. I had one for Nov-Jan very little 1-2 days. He said the injection has been known to stop or increase a woman's flow, but I don't know if that is the case here. It could have been from the trauma of the injury. I told him I would check with my doctor again. He then got into my pain level. He said what did Dr. Wake tell you about surgery? That he would never have to do surgery and to see you about injections. He said I see you had one and I would go on ahead and order the next one. I said for what? If my pain has not improved and the only thing the injection did was allowed me to sit down longer, why would I want another one. He said because you have had some improvement. I said, No. You treated my back based off the readings from a MRI in December.

I told him no one had requested another MRI to see why my lower back was burning, why my pain was radiating, and why I am having sharp pain? He said, Oh I can request another MRI. I said what happen to my EMG? He said, I can order that too. I gave you one injection in your L-5, but you are still having issues with your L4-S1. I can give you an injection for that.

He said, "Are you still on the Lyrica." I said, "No, you changed it due to side effects." You put me on Gabapentin. He said, "Oh yea that's right." How is it? I am still in pain and sharp pain while at work. He said, how many times a day? I said, "3 times a day." He said, "I am going to add another pill with that and see how it goes from there."

I told him I have a new doctor. I needed them to submit all my information to the new treating doctor. He said they could do that. He walked me to the front, told me to sit outside, and that he would be with me. I sat for a while and decided to walk back in and see why it was taking so long. Mick is a guy that works for him and he was filling out some paperwork.

He said, "Sign this." I said, what is that? Mick said, this is for the second injection. I said, "I am not signing that." Dr. Kai can speak to my doctor about all of this. Mick said Ok. I asked Dr. Kai, are you going to speak with my doctor about this? He said, "What is his name?" I spelled it for him and he said he is not in the system. I pulled out one of Dr. Stephens's card and he said, oh that's why I can't find him, he is a physician assistant. I asked if he was going to call him and fax everything over to him. He said, " Yes." I asked him what else I needed to do. He looked mad and said check out with the ladies at the desk.

I went to the front desk and she asked for my name. I gave it to her and she said, "Do you have a follow up with Dr. Kai?" I said, "I don't know, let me go ask him." I went back, his staff and him were huddled in the corner talking about Dr. Stephens. I asked did I have a follow up and he said, "No, I guess we will wait on your doctor. You will see him on Thursday anyway. I went back to the front desk to let them know I had a new doctor and would follow up with him.

On May 12, 2015, I sent my lawyer an email alerting her that Katherine from the insurance company called to schedule another MRI at an imaging clinic in Arlington. Little did I know that she and Vanessa (AOA W/C personnel) was assisting her with the locations for the MRI. I was asking about the EMG for the nerve damage to my back. I wrote my lawyer asking her: Why are they avoiding the EMG? I also let her know about the pain and burning in my lower back that radiates to my right hip.

Katherine and Vanessa got the MRI approved quickly because they are all working together. The MRI was scheduled for the next day 3:30 pm on Matlock in Arlington.

On May 13, 2015, I came to Central Imaging in Arlington, Texas. They still had Dr. Kai listed as my physician. They were going to send all my MRI results to him when my treating doctor had changed to Dr. Stephens.

I sent my lawyer an email and let her know what happen at the imaging clinic. My life has been on hold for 6 months with them. I am ready to move on.

My lawyer updated me on the W/C protocol. Your doctor makes the referrals and they usually have their own facilities they like to refer their patients too.

On May 14, 2015, I received a voicemail from Vanessa (Arlington Orthopedics Assoc.) today.

She left a voicemail saying: "On your last visit with Dr. Kai, he ordered 3 tests to be performed for you. One was for a repeat MRI, an EMG, and an ESI. I am calling to let you know the MRI was approved, but your WC insurance uses a service that contracts with different MRI facilities. They will be setting that MRI up and calling you. I am calling you because I won't know when and where you will have the MRI done. You will know before I will so when you hear from them with that appointment information, I need you to call me, so I can schedule you a follow up with Dr. Kai.

Deception of lies are listed below

1. Vanessa was working with the insurance company to locate the MRI Imaging place for me. The lady that called me on Tuesday said she was working with Vanessa to locate an office.

2. The office was located 5 blocks from Dr. Wake and Dr. Kai's office.

3. I put on the paperwork yesterday at the imaging place that I wanted my paperwork to go to Dr. Stephens and they sent it to Dr. Kai.

4. The clerk and staff at the imaging place were already briefed on how to handle me.

5. Dr. Kai told me during my first consultation with him that it would be an act of congress to get a second injection. Now, suddenly, he can get everything done.

6. I told Dr. Kai during my last visit about all the side effects and he says that the injection might have stopped my menstrual cycle.

7. If my diagnosis has been unchanged in areas, gotten worse, and have new medical issues that have appeared due to it taking so long, why would Dr. Kai and I need to revisit?

8. Dr. Kai placed me on Sertraline which made me so confused. I took it for two days and stopped. It began to slur my speech. It caused things to move in slow motion. Be careful of the drugs they prescribe for you and please watch out for side effects. If you put on any of the paperwork that your social time with people changed due to your injury, they assume that you are withdrawing from people. Keep people around you because you need their support during this time in your life.

10 – THE LIES BEGIN

On May 28, 2015, I received a letter from Broadspine approving me for three hours of therapy and one hour of psychiatric therapy concerning my pain. They also sent a letter for the approval of my EMG. I took everything to Wolmint today. Dr. Stephens said they would pay me four hours for therapy and four hours to work light duty. Dr. Felipe (My W/C Psychiatrist) said they were only going to pay me four hours. I would go to group therapy with the rest of the injured workers and we would discuss how to manage day to day while living in pain. We did several sessions which included meditation. Because our faith some of us choose not to close our eyes and breathe. We would do an assessment weekly or bi-weekly to discuss if we needed assistance with everyday activities, how was our attitude while dealing with the injury, video watching of others that had been injured and their recent updates, etc.

On June 5, 2015, I went to therapy and did the weekly testing. For some strange reason Jennifer put down that I lifted 40lbs off the floor during our initial visit. I told the head physical therapist (Teddy) that what she documented was incorrect. I attempted to lift it from the floor and it hurt my back. The calculations she showed were all wrong because she used a machine that they said didn't work. Teddy was explaining to Jennifer that the numbers she recorded were not correct and a normal healthy person could not do those numbers. She also didn't put my pain level down with each of those testing segments. We would test once a week. We would sit and do lunch with the entire work hardening group and the head therapist. I was determined that I would finish the work hardening program because I was committed.

I was doing the work hardening program and working a half a day. There was another employee name Nomarshall that had hurt his back on the job performing a different task. He was sent to me, so I could train him on what I was doing for light duty. Little did they know, he had a sister that was in human resources and knew the law. Nomarshall had herniated disc and nerve issue with his lower lumbar. After I trained him on what I was doing, he was able to work on one end as I worked on the opposite end of the production module. I missed some days due to my back and when I came back to work he was gone. The job could no longer accommodate his work restrictions and released him from light duty. Shortly after this happen they release me from light duty because my restrictions could not be accommodated any longer. This was because of this young man challenging their light duty procedures and followed up with his sister who was in Human Resources for another company.

I had a follow up with Dr. Stephens and he was pushing for another injection in my lower back or to try nerve burning with Dr. Miles. When I came in for my follow up visits with Dr. Stephens, he had not even checked my file and read the recent EMG findings. I asked him questions about the EMG and he was stumbling over the readings. I could see early signs with this clinic that it was equal too if not worse than Ova Medical. I sent my lawyer and email to check on North Texas Spine Clinic for me. I sent the results of my MRI to them and they said I was a candidate for their program. Wolmint was trying to manage my pain level.

On June 9, 2015, I met with all the doctors during their meeting to discuss surgery as my next line of treatment and Dr. Stephens said he would follow up with me. Several weeks went by and I still had no appointment for consultation set up with a neurosurgeon. I also gave them the information about North Texas Spine Clinic. The head Doctor over the facility ask for Stephens to follow up with the request and get back with me. I went to two follow ups with Dr. Stephen after this meeting and he still had not made any calls.

On June 12, 2015 I sent an email to my lawyer to bring her up to speed about everything that was going on at the new clinic. I was questioning my lawyer about contacts at the State Board Insurance concerning the treatment patients were receiving at the W/C clinics. I was at a new clinic listening to the horror stories of botched surgeries, denial of treatments, long waits for surgeries, missing paperwork, etc.

My lawyer said, Complaints regarding the carrier and worker's injury those typically go to your state representative as they are the governing body of the system. She was not able to look up the information for me, because their system was down.

On June 13, 2015, I finally received the report from Dr. Lamb, and he mentioned the removal of disc. I asked my lawyer the following questions. Can you help me get some resolution to move forward with surgery? She told me to mention what I sent her to Dr. Stephens and go from there.

I received a letter in the mail the following week for an appointment with Dr. Coleman for a RME (Required Medical Exam) on 24th of June at 11 am. This is a test ordered by the insurance company? This examination is for the insurance doctor to counter what the FCE (State Doctor) is saying about your injury and treatment.

On June 24, 2015, the company's insurance sent me to Dr. Coleman. The doctor did not have my previous MRI or EMG that was performed during the month of May and June. Dr. Coleman said, "I know you have probably been though one of these before?" I said, "Yes, I have."

He looked at a piece of paper and began to read off what he needed to exam me for. He said someone didn't agree with what the previous doctor said. He asked, "Did he side with you?" I said, "Yes he did." I gave him my updated information and he said don't pay any attention to that MRI or EMG report because they are not always accurate.

He asked where my pain was. I showed him my lower back and how the pain radiates around to the front. He said anything else? I told him about the tingling from around my back, right leg, both feet, numb toes on the right foot. He had me to sit on the exam table and he tapped below my knees. He said something was going on because I had no reflexes below my knees on both legs. It didn't show on my MRI report. He then asked for me to lie on my back. I asked him, "Do I need to lie on my back, because it hurts?" He said, "Yes, because what I have to check you for, I will need you on your back." He measured my thighs and the length from knee to ankle. He raised my foot up and asked if it hurts. I told him no for the left side, but yes, for the right foot. He then asked for me to lie on my stomach. He said, "Where does it hurt?" I took my hand and showed him where the pain radiates from. He pressed down next to my butt and spine. I told him that hurt. He said the medical term for the location of the pain, and I asked him, what does that mean? He said you have pain in your pelvic area. I said, "It's my L4-5. He said you don't even know where your L4-5 is. I showed him again and he said you are just repeating what everyone else has said. I said, "Well what about the EMG with 90% nerve damage." He said it may or may not be accurate and you are not going to die. We doctor are surgeons and we hardly ever use EMGs, they are for the insurance companies. He said, "You don't need surgery, what you need is another Epidural injection in your sciatic nerve and 8 more weeks of Work Hardening and you should be prepared to go back to work. I said, "Would you like a copy of my job duties?" He said, "No, hold on to that." I said what about the issue with my bone rubbing? He said those are tendons. I asked him how long will it take for me to heal? He said, "I don't know, you will heal, and you are a victim of an injury and this is not the end of the world."

I walked away from that clinic praying for this battle with my back and the insurance company to be over with. I was hurt, disappointed, and frustrated with this doctor's visit.

I didn't know anything else to do, but to email my lawyer and ask her the questions below:

1. Was this doctor picked by Worker's Injury or the company's insurance?
2. How long is this going to take?
3. Do you share information I send to you with the insurance company?
4. What does this look like at the end of this process?
5. Is he paid to report back what the insurance wants to hear?
6. What is my hope in this being resolved?
7. Who can I write to about this doctor and the treatment I received?
8. Was I supposed to be in the examiner room by myself with him?
9. How can he say, I can report back to work, and not look or study my chart prior to seeing me?
10. He never took the copy of my job descriptions that I tried to hand him.

How would he know what my back could tolerate?

On June 26, 2015 my lawyer answered all the questions above:

1. Insurance company
2. 10 days
3. No, but they have access to your medical records
4. You get rated for the injury you sustained once you are ready to be (meaning there is no further treatment anticipated to help you get better)
5. Basically
6. To have the judge side with the state designated doctor
7. Medical board
8. Yes, that's not an issue typically
9. Based on his exam of you
10. Based on his exam of you

Keep in mind this is the Insurance Carrier's doctor. All this is expected.

On June 26, 2015, one of the lawyers emailed me: I am requesting a conference on the back pay owed to you. I previously sent the carrier your earnings through 5-16-15, and though she did respond and said she'd review that, she's not responded since. It's my understanding the employer will no longer accommodate.

Monifa is working on getting full income benefits reinstated. In the meantime, can you please provide me with copies of all your check stubs. If you want to simply provide an updated payroll history, as you'd printed online before, that will be fine.

Lawyer: Tanya, we still want them to pay what's owed. I've requested a conference as they never got back on the partial benefits while you were working and earning less. Monifa has been working on getting benefits reinstated, but we just learned I believe around 6-22 that you weren't working, and now I understand you are going back again through 7-14-15? We want you paid, and I believe they're about to pay, but there are no guarantees, and if you're back at work light duty again we'll need to continue to get the post-injury check stubs to determine what's owed.

My lawyer explains the payout after missing days below:

Without missing consecutive days, you would not be owed any worker's injury, however, if you were making less on light duty than you were used to making then you would be owed the difference up to 70% for that period. Also, I need to confirm you were working on light duty and not full duty. Finally, I would need your check stubs to prove you were making less during this time.

Myself: Who protects my job through this process if Dr. Stephens (doctor at Wolmint) said go back since you are not protected? Tom (Night senior manager) said don't come back until they get your back taken care of? I am confused. Do I not go back since the system shows me on Leave or do I go to protect my job? I am willing to do as you say. Let me know, please?

Lawyer: That's a tough question to answer. The best answer that I can give you is that if your doctors say you are capable of working, and the employer will accommodate your restrictions, then you can go back. There are no guarantees about your job, whether you are working or not. The law says they cannot terminate you in retaliation for filing your Work Injury claim. It doesn't say that they must hold your job for you. If they were to let you go, they wouldn't say it's because you got hurt and we're mad about it. Our goal is to get you fixed, and get you compensated. We'd love you to be able to go back to doing what you were doing and make the same type of wages. I cannot guarantee you that will happen. So, if your employer can accommodate, and your doctors tell you it's ok, then it's ok.

Myself: I will talk to Tom on Sunday before I clock in. Do you know if they will fix my back or do I live with it as is? There is no way I can ever do my normal job function with my current state.

On June 29, 2015, from the lawyer: Tanya, any treatment issues would be related to either an extent of injury dispute, or a dispute as to the reasonable and necessary nature of the treatment that is being requested. Monifa is addressing these issues and I've copied her on this email. I'm working on the benefits owed. They are obligated to provide all reasonable and necessary treatment to the compensable injury, so any dispute would therefore be based upon either the treatment not being reasonable and medically necessary, or not related to what they've accepted. Monifa should be able to explain further. In the meantime, we'll still work on getting you paid.

My lawyer responds: Ms. Nelson, the adjuster wants to know if your employer gave you any written notification that they do not have light duty work for you? Please respond ASAP, I tried calling you but only got your voice message. Regarding treatment, your claim is accepted, treatment is not affected by the stop of pay so yes, the treatment is reasonable and necessary but other than that it will get approved.

Myself: I had an appointment with Dr. Stephens after therapy today. That's how I missed responding back timely. They do have light duty. Tom said for me not to come back until they got my back taken care of. He was not at work last night. If he is there today I will have him to write a statement and fax it over to you. I asked, Dr. Stephens to take me off work but he said I would have to do 8 hours of work hardening which is not helping me. I told him I was at a catch 22 because my back is not better, and you want me to do 8 hours of work hardening or continue 4 hours of work and 4 hours of work hardening. Dr. Stephen shrugged his shoulders with a lack of concern and said it's up to you.

11 – THE LETTER THAT CHANGED EVERYTHING

Another injured worker and myself began working on letters to send out to the White House, OSHA, Rainbow Coalition, Texas Department of Insurance, Our State Representatives, Congressmen and Congresswomen, Al Sharpton, Radio, Talk Shows, etc. We placed them in the mail and awaited a response from anyone that would help. What is in the letter below is what I went through in a one-year time span, and some of it is a repeat of what you have already read.

To Whom It May Concern:

I know we have more crucial things going on in America that are far more important than the issues with the Worker's Injury System. I know some people have taken advantage of the system, but I am not one of them. I have never had a work injury in my life in the 20 years of being in the workforce, until now. I injured my lower back (L4-5, S-1) on the job emptying a trash gondola. I went to the company's doctor, thinking they would do the right thing and now find myself in the old cliché, "don't go to your company's doctor because they are not going to do right by you." Well, I am living the cliché and I have witnessed so much that is wrong within the Worker's Injury Clinics, doctors, and the insurance companies.

During the first 6 months of my injury which occurred on 11-2-14, this was my experience

1.   The work restrictions that I received never were explained by the treating doctor. (Ova's physician - Dr. Stan and Dr. Britain -Wolmint-Dr. Stephens). No one explained because, so many people like myself, assume that the hours on the restrictions mean 2 hours work/15-minute break/2 more hours of work/30-minute lunch/ 2 hours of work/and a final 15-minute break.   My restrictions/body mechanics were not explained to me until December 2014 by my physical therapist at Ova.

2.   The physical therapist has a time frame in which they must get you back to work. My physical therapist would increase the weight lifting exercise immediately, instead of gradually working you up to the next level. For example, if you lift 10lbs today, well your body should be ready the next day or two for 15-20lbs. I gave Ova, Wolmint, and the first designated doctor a copy of my job descriptions with weight details noted on the

sheets. The RME doctor didn't want to know my job descriptions, but stated, I would be fit in 8 weeks to return to work with an injection and work hardening.

3.   My pain increased due to lifting a 40lb box weight at therapy. I was hesitating and told the therapist "No!" She insisted and reluctantly complied. This sent me to the ER at the end of Nov. 2014. My pain elevated with a vengeance and with burning in my lower back.

4.   It took 3 weeks of burning and pain before my first MRI was administered. I got the first MRI on December 12, 2014. After they completed the MRI it took 2 weeks before they read it to me. The clinic said they never received it and the imaging center said they sent it the next day.

5.   I continued to work in pain daily while on prescription meds. The workers injury doctor purposely schedules you a month later for follow-up, to keep you at work if possible. When you are taken off work they might schedule to see you every 2 weeks.

6.   Insurance companies are dictating to the doctors what the injured employee will or will not receive. They are in it to make money for the business. They can care less about the injured worker.

7.   Patients doing therapy for 6 months or more and still show no or very little improvement with their injury. They are tested bi-weekly for improvement. The test consists of lifting, flexing, carrying, and stepping for 10 seconds - 3 minutes for each test interval. Does this test justify that a person can do their normal job task for 8 or more hours?

8.   Why is scheduling done a month out or later before something is done to help? Do you think an injured worker's injuries increases while on light duty or decreases?

9.   Why are injured employees sent through multiple surgeries before the insurance approves therapy? This allows scar tissue to settle which causes a second surgery.

10.   During the time of injury all the employee's time off is used up and worker's injury never reimburses their pay.

11.   Appointments are set at a time where you must drive great distance, during your work shift, which causes you to lose pay.

12.   Things are purposely put off frustrating the injured employee, so they will give up. Because of the long wait, new medical issues arise due to stress and waiting.

13.   Instead of dealing with the injury, they drug you up with medicine. You go to work for 8 hours, and then attend 4-6 months of therapy for 2 hours a day. Is this fair to the injured worker?

15.   Who do you really have in the worker's injury system that is for the injured employee?

16.   Why does Worker's Injury do everything to rule in favor of the employer? Are the doctor's given incentives to side with the insurance companies? On several occasions someone keyed my social security information incorrectly; then I'm not allowed to change doctors because I did not have a good cause. During that time, they were waiting on the report from the first designated doctor Dr. Lamb.

17.   They denied my request to change treating doctors three times before my requests were approved. I now have approval, but they're still sending my insurance information to the old doctor. Why?

18.   The orthopedic doctor said I could return to work lifting 25lbs after my first epidural injection on February 9, 2015. I got an attorney who has done very little in my case, but collect money from Worker's Injury for the little help they have provided.

20. I feel I was used as an experiment when something didn't work. I was placed on medicine that made me dizzy, confused, off-balance, not able to comprehend much around me. Now they have me, along with others, seeing a psychiatrist for our pain. It's not in my head, it's my back, hip, and lower right stomach.

19. Worker's Injury rules are updated frequently to side with the employers.

20. While testing at the new clinic, the therapist wrote down false numbers to get me in the program for work hardening. The equipment used to test me was not working properly. The clinic is paid $800-$1704 per work injury for work hardening. Everyone is being paid well, but the injured worker finds no resolution.

21. On June 24, 2015 the company's insurance sent me to another
designated doctor appointment at 4222 Trinity Mills in Dallas, Texas to
see Dr. George Cookman. The doctor did not have my previous MRI
or EMG that was performed during May and June. Dr. Cookman said,
"I know you have probably been though one of these before." I said,
"Yes I have." He looked at a piece of paper and began to read off what
he needed to exam me for. He said, "Someone didn't agree with what
the previous doctor said, did he side with you?" I said, "Yes he did."

I gave him my updated information and he said, "Don't pay any attention
to that MRI or EMG report because they are not always accurate." He
asked me, "Where are you in pain?" I showed him my lower back and told
him the pain radiated around to the front. He asked, "anything else? "I told
him about the tingling from my back around, right leg, both feet, numb
toes on the right. He had me to sit on the exam table and tap below my
knees.

He then asked for me to lie on my back. I asked him to do I need to lie on
my back, because it hurt. He said "Yes, because what I have to check for is
I need you on your back." He measured my thighs and the length from
knee to ankle. He raised my foot up and asked if it hurts. I told him yes,
with the right foot. He then asked for me to lie on my stomach.

He said where does it hurt? I took my hand and showed him where the
pain radiates from. He pressed down next to my butt and spine. I told him
that hurt. He said "the medical term for the location of the pain. It was my
pelvic area." I said it's my L4-5 and he said, "you don't even know where
your L4-5 is." I showed him again and he said, "You are just repeating what
everyone else has said." I said, "Well what about the EMG with 90% nerve
damage?" He stated, "It may or may not be accurate and you are not going
to die, "We doctors are surgeon and we hardly ever use EMGs, they are for
the insurance companies." He said, "You don't need surgery, what you
need is another Epidural injection in your sciatic nerve and 8 more weeks
of Work Hardening and you should be prepared to go back to work." I
said, "Would you like a copy of my job duties?" He said, "No hold on to
that." I said, what about the issue with my bone rubbing? He said, that was
your tendons, you will heal, and you are a victim of an injury and this is not
the end of the world."

I walked away from that clinic praying for this battle with my back and
the insurance company to be over with. I was hurt, disappointed, and
frustrated. My back is in a tug-a-war, but I find strength in standing for

what is right and I reflect on the people that have been suffering longer than I.

I have gone through different treatments and I am back at square one. The only thing I can do is sit a little while longer. The horror stories you hear when it comes to people at the clinics are heart breaking. I have realized several things since my injury:

A. I will never look at an injured person and judge them on their injury.

B. I never want to be in a position where money, numbers, or safety percentages rules over the quality of life for an individual.

C. I know how it feels to watch others in pain.

D. I have experienced nothing. My house notes got behind for almost two months, I had a friend and family that gave me money for food and gas, my old boss and her daughter paid all my utility bills.

E. I would like for my back to receive proper treatment. I would like for Worker Comp to reimburse me for all the day's pay I have missed.

F. I would like for someone to come in and speak with some of the injured workers without retaliation or fear of losing their benefits.

G. I would like for some of the rules in the Worker Injury system to be changed so there is correct medical treatment for the workers, proper therapy as it relates to the injured worker's job duties, and W/C pay to start without delay, so the injured worker can still provide for their family.

H. I am told by the second designated doctor to ignore the MRI and EMG, but he said,

"You have not reflexes below your knees, but it's not showing on the MRI report."(???)

There are layers in this onion (Worker's Injury system) that needs to be peeled back and exposed for what it is. I placed some of my journey behind this letter, but there are so many more people that are suffering at the hands of this system. They are choosing to make themselves worse to provide for their families and others are going along with the doctors to get a check.

This system places numbers over the health and quality of life for an injured employee that was doing a job at the time of his/her injury. This is a system where people are tired, frustrated, and wounded. I don't know if I am even sending this to the correct person, but I am stepping out on faith that someone will have a heart to hear my cry and answer the call for change. I speak on behalf of the people that are going through the same thing, but with different body parts. I also fear for the next generation that will have to deal with this. Somewhere the system was broken and somewhere the system needs to be fixed.

I forward this letter out to my lawyer on July 22, 2015, by saying, I sent this letter out on the 26th of June and the young lady at the Texas Worker's Injury department asked for me to send this to you. She is getting calls from
Texas Congressman office to report back to them. I also got a call on Monday from Texas Department of Insurance. I told her to expect calls from about 12 more people. She (TWC) clarified how things work and said
I am being handled like a ping pong ball. She asked for me to stay in contact with her. I will send you the list of organizations I sent it to also.

My lawyer's response to the letter:
 Ms. Nelson, I read the letter and thankfully I read your subsequent email, we have done nothing but work tirelessly to get you paid, treated, and better since we started on the case. I understand the frustration with worker's injury but when my ability to do my job is questioned I am dismayed when I have been in constant contact with you as to status and developments as they happen. If in the future you have an issue with me please let me know so I can address it, if you have questions, ask them, we are here to help you not hurt you. We are the only ones in the process who want your claim to do well since we are directly dependent on that being so for us to receive any type of benefit. It's in MY best interest to make sure you are happy, healthy, and paid. Have a good day.

My reply to them (lawyer), I understand what you are saying, and I apologize again. I just want this over with already. I am with this almost one year and I want normalcy again. Thank you all for what you are doing for me.

DEEPER INTO THE BATTLE, BUT FINALLY RELIEF

I am deeper into the battle because my job is up in the air, I have sent letters out for someone to consider the Work Injury System, I have another clinic that is not providing decent medical treatment for my back, and I have ticked my lawyers off who has been of help to me. What do I do now? I text my night senior manager about whether to come in and he responded back via text. I had filed for disability through my job and it was denied. I couldn't get the worker's injury doctors to release me from work. My Night Senior noticed how I was pushing just to get through the night and said they could not accommodate my work restrictions any longer. I also told him about my pay that was still short and his response below.

Tom: Did you come in yesterday?

Tanya: Yes, can you call me?

Tom: I am getting on a flight will call u later.

Tanya: Ok, they denied my benefits while I was out for FMLA and short-term disability. They won't pay me for the days I missed concerning my back. I explained to them that you told me not to come back until my back was situated. I called HR and they were processing everything like it was a go, but they sent me the denial letter on last Wednesday. My lawyer is asking for you to write a statement and then Tam will release my payment. They have not paid me all month for the 4 hours of therapy or for last week. I am short $1200 this month for bills.

Tom: Tanya, what dates are we talking about?

I remember telling you they were required to pay you while you were going thru therapy and for you to come in for part of the shift. Wanda (HR Manager) communicated to me to tell you not to report back to work. I am not understanding what they are challenging

Tanya: The week of the June 15-16-17,2015 When I called off and was trying to make the last day.

Tom: I will contact her Tuesday to see what she needs. I will get with you after that.

Tanya: I went in last night because Aetna said I had not reached my anniversary to take off FMLA. Sorry about texting you. Tam has held up all my funds and I have not paid my mortgage for June. Bones are rubbing in back, hip is hurting, right leg and both feet tingling, toes numb, and this is acceptable? I don't mind the battle but when I am being mistreated, my health is being jeopardized, and something must give. The doctor never said after you finish the treatment they would pay you he said I would be paid. Sorry about venting but this is my back I am fighting for.

On July 2, 2015, I went to the Ortho visit at Wolmint yesterday. I told Dr. Wills I would like to consult with the neurosurgeon. Dr. Wills was speaking with me about another epidural injection. I let him know I was interested in meeting with a neurosurgeon. While going in for work hardening during the week, I would ask the front desk or my therapist about a CT scan on my back. The therapist told me to follow up with the doctor. I made several friends that shared their stories and experiences while being in this clinic. There were people that worked for federal and state government businesses. People had several surgeries, 7-15 injections, and therapy, but wasn't better. The front desk clerk dismissed me from the program. I asked Lacy to give me a copy of the email, so I could fax it to my lawyer. When she gave it to me, I read the correspondence about me getting more therapy but nothing beyond that. I left the premises heading home. There was a young lady that was about to commit suicide on HWY 67. I had gotten pass her before I realized what was going on. I called 911 and had her to stay on the phone with me until I drove back around. I got on the wrong entrance and told the 911 dispatcher I would call her back. I begin to pray for the young lady and when I made it back around where she was, another lady was talking her down and asking her to live for her kids. My issues seemed small compared to her and I was glad Yahweh saved her that day.

Mid July I begin preparing for a BRC (Benefit Review Conference) hearing. I received letters from the insurance lawyers about my treatment from beginning to current. I read some of the doctors' statements and was blown away with their lies. They hardly ever touched my back, but gave their diagnosis off their own view point of me.

August 28, 2015,

I went to the doctor's appointment today and Dr. Stephens was reading my EMG report that was done 2 months ago. He also said that my blood work came back from last month and it had contents of sugar in it. I needed to see my primary doctor about my blood sugar levels. I told him they didn't take blood from me, only urine. He said, "Oh they didn't." "I said, "No only urine." He said, "Oh we had someone else's specimen information in your file." I told him, "You tested my urine last month and you are testing it again." He said, "The urine test last month was for the insurance company and the urine test this month is for me." I knew he was not being truthful. If someone's paperwork was mixed in with mine, who else has been treated like this. I told Dr. Stephens, I wouldn't let them do my blood work anymore and I would go to my primary doctor who I trust. He looked at me and I at him. I begin to pray for him and he said, what did you say?" I said, " I am praying for you." He said, I pray for my patients all the time, I told him not to pray for me because I did not know who he was praying too. Each time I had to check out at the front desk, I would have to wait and have the paperwork redone. They would put the wrong wording down. After I receive my paperwork and medication, we left.

My aunt asked, "Do you always have to wait so long to be seen?" I replied, "Yes." She said, "Do they mix people's lab results up often?" I told her, I don't know, but good question. She said, "He was not dressed like a doctor and he was not professional at all." I said, "He dress like that some time, and he was trying to argue with me about my blood work." My aunt said, "Go to YELP and file a complaint and with the medical board."

I filed a complaint against Dr. Stephens with the insurance company and on YELP. They did not let me see Dr. Stephens after this complaint was filed.

12 – CLOSING

My lawyer called and said my hearing with the BRC had been cancelled and they were going to send me a check for my back pay for benefits. She said, "Let me know when you receive it." She later called back and said to keep the appointment because you need to sign some paperwork and I will be on the phone, along with their lawyer, and a mediator. I did receive a check along with two more after that. I knew the battle was not over.

When I received the checks, I owe money out to friends and family that helped pay my bills during this crucial time. I got everything caught up around the house. The insurance company began to send my Worker's injury check late which put me behind on my mortgage. I notified my lawyer of what was going on. They got in contact with the adjuster and she began to release my checks on time again. When you notice there is some form of retaliation done under handily, you must alert someone quickly.

Remember you will never have one battle at a time but multiple ones at the exact time. My new level of elevation is Dr. Wills at the clinic. I see him once a month and normally they already know what treatment I will receive.

I don't sit longer than 30-37 minutes now. I am called back to have my weight taken, blood pressure, and temperature checked. After there is a series of questions about your pain level and urine test every two months.

1. What is your pain? Is that with or without medicine? What will it be without medicine?

2. What helps to reduce your pain?

3. What makes it worse?

4. How is your sleep?

5. Are you still taking the following medications?

Once this person leaves he/she goes and give the doctor an update on your status. I am going through this repeatedly. I started herbs during the summer to see if it would help with the inflammation and pain. I continue to take them along with some powder herb for relaxation. The herbs are not bad on your liver and kidney. I weaned myself off all the prescription drugs to see how much impact they really had on my back. I am still experiencing the same symptoms I have been having while on all those drugs. As of 2016, my lower back has pain, burning, sharp pain, tingling, and when I am walking, it feels like bones rubbing together, my right hip/

groin area bothers me, tingling down my right leg and both feet, numbness of toes on my right foot, pain and spasm periodically on my right lower stomach. I am still going back and forth about the treatment for my back.

The insurance has denied my request for a standing and sitting MRI and my next doctor's appointment is at the end of January 2016. I don't trust that they would even do the right thing for my back now. I receive poor treatment from physical therapy with the box weight. I received an injection that never should have been given when surgery should have been performed.

I got a clinic that would rather keep me drugged and injected up to suppress the pain instead of dealing with my injury. I wrote this book, so you can know you are not alone during this process. You also have more rights than you know, and you don't have to live in fear. I would love for the people who put the laws or rules in place for Worker's Injury to come back to the table and start all over. It would bring me great joy for journalist to go into the clinics and interview some of their previous patients and the patients that have filed complaints about their medical treatment in the past.

When Yahweh says, "I AM....Bigger than Your Worker's Injury, He Really Is."

ABOUT THE AUTHOR

I have been a writer for most of my adult life. However, when I was younger, I desired to be a teacher. I studied journalism in high school and loved it. I began writing in early 2000 about the things I was dealing with pertaining to life. My mom passed away 2007 and the zeal to write was gone.

Yahweh impressed upon my heart to write in 2011 and I started again. I wrote letters to inform people of what was going on in the work injury system, but got little help. He prompted me to release the first book, "I AM Bigger Than Your Work Injury."
    I love people and I know that is why I fight so hard for their silent voices to be heard.

As a mother of one, and engaged to my fiancé, Andrew, I look forward to impacting the nations of our world with the Good News.

Part Two: Torture Chamber- Legalize Bullying in America/Gas Lighting

Connect with me via social media!
- On Twitter: www.twitter.com/tanya0673
- **On Facebook:** www.facebook.com/tanya.nelson.3958
- Targeted Individuals United on Facebook